Intermittent Fasting Diet 101

Intermittent Diet Guide for Beginners - Women and Weight Loss

TABLE OF CONTENTS

INTRODUCTION

Weight loss is a challenging health and fitness goal. It is anchored on the desire to achieve well-being and greater self-esteem.

It can change lives and improve the way that we see the world. However, this is not an easy task. As proof, there have been countless dieting schemes and plans that people try and follow, but sometimes to no avail.

The dieting world is always coming up with novel ways to develop new diets, which people can try and follow for their success. But still, many dieters end up giving up their dieting and weight loss challenge because it is grueling and difficult.

There is a valid reason to this. Indeed, it is difficult to give up one of the best pleasures in life – food.

If only there can be a dieting scheme that will help people achieve weight loss while still enjoying their desired lifestyle and choice of food, it would spell out success for the lives of many.

Luckily, there is a dieting program that allows people to lose weight while still enjoying the best of their chosen lifestyle. This is known as *intermittent fasting.*

Fasting connotes hunger and restriction of food control, but intermittent fasting as a weight loss strategy does not imply this.

Intermittent fasting is one of the most effective, lifestyle-friendly, and easiest to follow diets out there.

True, there is a degree of challenge following this diet, but if you have access to the right strategies and best tips for this diet, the success would definitely outweigh any challenge or difficulty.

Would you like to lose weight and change your life? Have you always been overweight and feeling down about how you see yourself?

Then try intermittent fasting. If you are a beginner – whether of intermittent fasting or weight loss in general – you are lucky to have this book in your hands.

"Intermittent Fasting Diet 101" contains proven steps and strategies on how to use the intermittent fasting method to achieve the best health through optimum weight loss.

Written for beginners, it will tell you everything that you need to know and guide you through every step of your weight loss endeavor. You will never be confused about intermittent fasting and learn the right way to follow it.

In this book, you will learn about the following:

- The motivational reasons to lose weight and how to never lose the inspiration to keep on achieving your desired figure
- What intermittent fasting is all about – how it works, why is it popular, and why you should engage in it
- The three main methods of intermittent fasting and how you can easily incorporate it to your lifestyle
- The pros and the cons of each method to help you choose which one is the best for you
- So much more about weight loss and dieting tips

You will no longer have to worry about dieting as you learn about the intermittent fasting method.

This unique dieting regimen promises weight loss according to your expectations – and with minimal effort on your part.

You will learn how to control food consumption, listen to your body, and design a dieting plan that will work for you.

This means that you will still enjoy your favorite food! Intermittent fasting will let you control your cravings and help you manage your weight at the same time.

If you intend to change your lifestyle and achieve the weight loss that you desire, the following pages will serve as a pathway towards reaping the success of your chosen endeavor.

Thanks again for downloading this book, I hope you enjoy it!

Chapter 1

Why Lose Weight?

Weight loss is driving a multi-billion dollar industry that has been existing for decades.

This started in the modern era when manufactured and standardized goods were sold. People became aware of dress sizes, differences in their figures, and ultimately the spectrum from healthy to unhealthy was defined.

Advances in medicine asserted that there was a medical reason for weight loss, and what varying weights and figures signified in human health.

Since then, we acquired consciousness regarding our weight and figure. Weight loss became a boom, since we normally did not care about where the pin points on the weighing scale – most people were unhealthy voracious eaters.

The scale even became a household object around this period, when previously it had been used only for mundane things.

However, decades of pursuing weight loss did not exactly result to progress in general.

The industry continues to perfect itself and find novel ways. Weight loss is proven as a difficult ordeal and not easily achievable for everyone.

From weight loss pills and tea to surgery, losing weight has never been so complex and varied, if we think about the available methods.

Why are they constantly being developed and improved?

Why have we not yet discovered and implemented the perfect weight loss strategy, even after decades of research and practice?

Is there anything lacking in our science and technology?

But before we answer that, let's get to the root of the cause. Is there really a need to lose weight? Isn't weight loss just a product of modernity and industrialization?

Let's look at the medical side first, the most rational and logical side of the debate.

Keeping an optimal weight is rather a must, and this has been proven in medical researches. Excess weight can cause several health problems.

There is a long list of illnesses that one can get just because of some extra weight. Most of this is common knowledge. A short list includes the following:

- Hypertension
- Heart attacks
- Atherosclerosis (fat plaques that clog arteries)
- Diabetes
- Stroke
- Cancer

Weight loss and keeping the body weight within the optimum range can significantly reduce the risk for all these diseases and health problems.

In fact, even a small decrease in weight can already improve one's cholesterol levels, blood pressure and blood glucose levels.

The first answer to the question of the need to lose weight is simple: for better health. Everybody wants to achieve better health; without it, much of our human experience will be greatly limited.

Nevertheless, the benefits of losing weight go beyond physical health.

This is why even people at a normal weight range still keep watch of their weight and prevent any significant weight gain.

Moving from the medical perspective, let's look at the emotional and psychological component of weight loss.

Arguably, weight loss helps to gain better self-image and more confidence.

If not for medical reasons, people want to lose weight because it makes them feel great. Whether or not this is a positive point, we are judged by the world according to the weight that we carry.

This is not due to prioritizing looks over attitude. Definitely, our weight reflects our lifestyles, discipline, and what choices do we make as individuals.

On a daily basis, an ideal weight makes moving around much easier, too. It makes us more efficient as beings whose bodies and ways of life are designed for moving or exerting physical effort.

Here are some of the top benefits why you should start losing weight today, apart from what have been discussed in the previous paragraphs.

Better sleep

Sleep is a basic need. Losing sleep impairs cognitive functioning and the way we positively experience our lives.

According to medical researches, there is a connection between weight loss and the quality of sleep. If you intend to improve your sleeping lifestyle, it is good to start with weight loss.

According to a paper presented at a joint meeting of the Endocrine Society and the International Society of Endocrinology, obese people who lost at least 5% of their body weight were able to sleep better.

In short, weight loss or nearing ideal weight significantly improves how we experience sleep in our lives. Conversely, if we are not in our optimal weight, we compromise the quality of our sleeping lifestyle.

Better brain function

If you can have a more efficient brain and mind, why would you not opt to have it?

Aside from engaging in activities that stimulate the brain and improve our cognitive activities, weight loss can also be a key towards achieving better mental health and well-being.

A study conducted in 2013 found that obese participants posted lower scores on cognitive tests compared to their counterparts who had healthy weight.

A different study found out that obesity leads to weakening of the blood-brain barrier. What could be the connection? And what is the medical explanation behind this?

If you have a significantly high body fat percentage, more fat cells are allowed to flow and enter the brain.

These fat cells can clog the blood vessels supplying oxygen and nutrients to the brain. Impaired blood flow can cause poor brain function. These fat cells can also compete or interfere with brain function.

By losing weight and improving the fat profile in the body, better blood flow resumes. The brain is able to function better.

Better skin condition

Skin blemishes and problems are linked to obesity. Psoriasis and eczema, among other skin problems, are believed to stem from a complex chain reaction initiated by obesity.

The skin becomes more prone to develop infections and problems like eczema. Premature skin aging is also one negative effect of obesity to the skin.

Before you consult a dermatologist, you may first consider weight loss as a solution to the problem.

Increased fat deposits can lead to the release of hormones that cause hormonal imbalance in the body.

This can lead to the increased risk for the development of several skin problems. An excellent weight keeps your hormones regulated and likewise decreases the chances for the development of skin problems.

Better liver and intestinal function

The liver and the intestines are delicate internal organs of the body. Much of our physiological functioning depends on these organs.

If we can prevent factors, especially lifestyle choices, that may harm these organs, we must do so.

Obesity can cause problems with liver function and intestinal elimination. Conversely, an excellent weight will help you protect these organs better.

Obesity can lead to the buildup of toxins within the blood, which can get deposited to the skin layers.

Toxin accumulation can lead to poor skin health and integrity, as has been mentioned, and also affect liver and intestinal functioning.

Better productivity

The upside of a losing weight is better productivity. As we have mentioned, the body at an optimal weight is able to function more efficiently.

We are not just talking about ease of movement and better balance.

There is also less fatigue, better resistance against stress and more energy to accomplish additional tasks if we are in our optimal weight.

Productivity will of course affect the quality of your lifestyle. All of these better abilities can help one to earn more.

Obesity, on the other hand, interferes with productivity. Health problems related to excess weight can lead to low productivity, missed days at work, more sick days and short-term disability.

There is also the cost of medications and hospitalization, worker's compensation and other kinds of personal costs brought about by obesity and the health problems it causes.

Better joint health

Carrying too much weight strains the joints, most especially those in the knees, ankles and pelvis.

If your bones have been aching lately, this might be due to the extra weight that you carry. If you have a job that requires you to stand by for hours, these pains might be dangerous to your bones.

Chronic stress and pressure on the joints can lead to inflammatory processes in the body. This can lead to pain and disability. Losing weight, on the other hand, eases off a lot of the strain on the joints.

This reduces inflammation and pain. A study in Wake Forest University has found that symptoms of knee osteoarthritis significantly decrease by just losing 10% of the body weight. There is also better mobility an improved ambulation.

Better sexual health

Sexual health is a large component of a decent and satisfactory lifestyle.

Linking weight and figure to that aspect, there is more to achieving optimal weight than just looking attractive for partners or potential partners.

Obesity is not just about fat accumulation in the body.

It also affects hormones and sexual energy. One, excess weight reduces stamina for satisfying sexual activities. Two, hormonal disruptions related to obesity can decrease libido.

Three, obesity (in various capacities) can affect fertility. Four, obesity affects confidence and self-esteem, making one feel unattractive and un-sexy. By losing weight, all of these problems can be solved. You can achieve better sexual health not by reading magazines, but by focusing on weight loss and living up to your goals.

CHAPTER 2

What is Intermittent Fasting?
Benefits of this Weight Loss Method

In the last chapter, you have learned of all the reasons to lose weight, especially if you are obese.

We all want to achieve the benefits of weight loss. But why is it that some people stay obese, even when information such as in the last chapter is mostly common knowledge?

A simple answer is their lack of information regarding the most effective and efficient method of losing weight – intermittent fasting.

Of all the myriad of weight loss solutions, intermittent fasting is one of the most effective and least costly options. This method will not make you take diet pills or supplementary vitamins; it is not expensive.

This method is not a diet plan; it will not tell which and which you could not eat. It isn't about eliminating certain food groups or eating specially-prepared meals; you don't have to pine for foods that you have always enjoyed.

If intermittent fasting is completely unlike popular weight loss strategies such as consciously cutting calories and avoiding food groups, then what is it, exactly?

Intermittent fasting is all about eating patterns.

Other dieting plans have focused so much and what you should and should not eat, they lack the most essential (or even the only important) factor that you need to consider about dieting: eating patterns.

This is all about how you consume food, when, and what role does eating food constitute in your daily lifestyle.

As you will notice when you follow intermittent fasting, eating patterns constitute the real success of your diet.

Intermittent fasting does not put much focus on what you eat. Practitioners of intermittent fasting believe that eating is a basic human pleasure, and it should not be compromised for the sake of losing weight.

This dieting regimen simply requires careful planning of when to eat and when not to.

The goal is to eat at times when the body can get the most out of the food. This results to more efficient consumption of food, thrift, and most of all, self-discipline.

In contrast to other weight loss solutions, intermittent fasting is not about crash diet and restrictive eating.

Here you will not experience grueling pains and craving of food. It actually promotes eating in order to lose weight. At the start of the process, it is important to keep the calorie intake the same.

You may be shocked by this first rule, because all of the dieting schemes promotes less caloric intake.

On the other hand, you will be relieved, because you would never have to truly limit yourself and break from what you previously enjoyed.

How does this method work?

Intermittent fasting works by taking advantage of the body changes when it is in the "fed" state and when it is in the "fasted" state.

This is all about dieting in cooperation with what your body naturally undergoes. The goal is to promote maximum food and energy use in each of these states. You take advantage of what happens in your body and learn to listen to the rhythm of your physiology.

To understand how intermittent fasting works, take a look at what happens to the body. Let's look at the biological perspective.

The "fed state" refers to the condition after eating a meal. The body digests the food and eventually absorbs the nutrients.

This state typically begins when you start to eat and continues until 3 to 5 hours after. What occurs during these hours?

Digestion and absorption happens during 3 to 5 hours post prandial (after eating). The body uses energy from the digested food.

Insulin levels are also high because of the glucose absorbed from the intestines. There is very minimal fat burning going on during the fed state because of these conditions.

After food has been digested and the nutrients are absorbed by the blood, the body enters the post-absorptive state.

In this condition, glucose and other nutrients would have entered the cells. Insulin levels start to drop because there isn't much for it to do. The body, particularly the digestive system, is done with processing the meal.

This state generally lasts between 8 and 12 hours. After the post-absorptive state comes the "fasted state".

During the fasted state, energy from food is either used up or stored. The energy requirements to keep the systems functioning would now come from somewhere else.

In this state, the body is able to access fat stores and turn it into energy. Insulin levels are at their lowest, which supports burning fat for energy.

Here is the part where your body is actively burning fat – with or without exercise – and this is the part which intermittent fasting takes advantage of.

These alternating states – explained by science – are the basis for weight loss using the intermittent fasting method.

You can see clearly where weight loss happens during this process. It occurs in the state where your body *naturally* burns fat.

The body is allowed to eat anything during the fed state. It does not matter whether you feast on high-carb, low-carb, high-fat, or low-fat meals – they are merely seen as sources of energy which your body needs.

Discipline or self-control is implied because you will naturally feel full after a meal. You cannot overeat during the feeding window because your body can simply not permit this.

Ample time is then given to enter a fasted state. Here you stop consuming food so that your body efficiently burns fat together with your previously consumed calories.

There is no need to change what people eat, how they eat, or how much food they eat. What is only being given focus here is the eating pattern.

The amount of exercise is also not a huge factor because the main target is on stimulating fat burning during the fasted state.

This is again, a natural process, something that your own body is capable of with minimal effort or intervention from you.

Most people who eat according to the "normal eating pattern" (i.e., eating every after few hours) fail to take advantage of the fat burning cycle during the fasted state. Note that this fat burning state is achieved 12 hours after a meal.

Most people do not have this much time in between meals. Hence, their bodies are used to relying more on energy from food rather than from burned fats.

If you can re-focus your body towards burning fat for energy, you will eventually lose fat and reach your targeted weight – all because you consumed food according to the appropriate pattern.

Benefits of Intermittent Fasting (IF)

There are many benefits to gain with intermittent fasting. It is not limited to efficient fat burning and weight loss.

Intermittent fasting can even be considered a lifestyle improvement. There are several benefits to intermittent fasting that you could not associate with other dieting schemes.

Intermittent Fasting (IF) simplifies the day.

Unlike most weight loss regimens, IF helps make your day much simpler. Other diets will make you prepare special food and meals in order to meet the dietary requirements.

There are even diets that make you prepare several small meals every day!

In IF, there is no need to prepare complex meals or count calories. All you have to do in order to jumpstart your day and stimulate fat burning is to drink a glass of water.

Nothing could be easier than that – no work outs and sweating tons from hard labor.

On an additional note, you get to reduce the time that you spend for preparing meals. You can live a minimalist lifestyle with no worries if you follow IF.

There is no need for planning, shopping and preparing 3 meals in a day (in some diets, about 5 to 6 different meals).

With IF, you get to worry about 1 less meal for each day, or more, depending on the type of IF you are following.

This is a very convenient eating pattern to follow and you can do more activities when you spend less time eating and worrying about what you eat.

IF prolongs life

Weight loss itself is key to prolonging our life span. But did you know that your dieting scheme can also improve and prolong your life?

IF has this certain advantage over other dieting schemes. The bodily processes that occur during fasting have an effect on our immunity and preservation systems.

Several researches support the concept that calorie restrictions can help in prolonging life.

The idea behind this is the fact that the body has intrinsic self-preservation mechanisms. Starvation (or fasting) triggers these mechanisms and the body seeks ways to prolong life.

However, with IF, there is no need to starve yourself. But you can achieve the same benefits that starvation provides through IF.

Self-preservation and healing can occur in your body. The steps in IF trigger the same mechanisms that starvation does to initiate the body's life-prolonging processes.

IF can reduce certain cancer risks

Awareness of cancer and its widespread occurrence should make us prioritize lifestyle strategies that would help us avoid it. IF can in fact reduce the risks of cancer, adding another advantage to this unique dieting scheme.

However, as much as more researches in cancer still need to be conducted, this benefit of IF regarding reducing cancer risk still needs more research results to back it up.

However, early researches found very promising results that link IF to cancer risk reduction.

One study has even found reduced chemotherapy side effects when patients went into intermittent fasting during cancer treatments.

Another study has found that going on IF during cancer treatments result in faster and improved cure rates and reduced cancer death rates.

These researches prove that there is a link between cancer and IF. Hopefully this connection can make us think of ways in which IF could be considered an aid to cancer or an addition to cancer treatment.

IF is so much easier to follow and maintain than traditional dieting

The patterns of eating and the behavior associated with it are the true reasons of obesity. If a person had better eating patterns and control when it comes to eating, obesity can be definitely prevented.

Obesity as a medical condition is in fact a behavioral problem. IF believes that weight gain and difficulty with weight loss is a matter of behavior.

Obesity is not about eating the wrong foods or eating in the wrong amounts. These matters are supposed to be controlled by our natural appetite and feelings of fullness. Most people start a diet or weight loss regimen on a high note.

Food consumption is controlled according to type or quantity. Usually, a plateau is reached – the stopping of initial weight loss – and then everything goes downhill.

IF is an easy lifestyle to follow. There are no food or calorie restrictions. You can eat anything, as much as you want.

This leaves you feeling good and not deprived. A pleasurable weight loss experience is more sustainable over a longer period rather than a strict, restrictive and exclusive one.

CHAPTER 3

Methods of Intermittent Fasting: Lean Gains

The Leangains method is one of the better known methods of intermittent fasting. This is also known as the 16:8 method.

It is popular among bodybuilders and those who intend to lose fat but pack muscle. It was designed by Martain Berkhan. This is also referred to as the daily intermittent fasting method.

Leangains is most recommended for people who are dedicated to gym workouts. It is great for losing body fat while building muscle mass.

The focus here is on body re-composition rather than the traditional weight loss or shedding off of pounds. Normally, people who go on Leangains for body re-composition end up with a heavier weight but with less fat.

How Leangains works

Leangains requires a 14-hour fast for women (16-hour fast for men) who want to lose fat and at the same time, build muscle.

The fasting-feeding cycle is done on a daily basis. If you apply this method, you have 14 or 16 hours of rest or doing any activity that you choose.

The remaining 6 to 8 hours of the day is spent on eating. Rather, these are the hours when you can freely consume food.

During the fast, there should be no calorie intake from food. This is the number one rule of intermittent fasting.

Beverages are permitted, which includes diet soda, calorie-free sweeteners, and black coffee.

Sugar-free gum is also allowed during the fasting period. What's important here is to stop the intake of a significant number of calories that are acquired from a normal serving of food.

The hours in which you should hold the fasting and the feeding period are entirely up to you. You can adapt this method according to your lifestyle.

When do you usually eat? What meals can be skipped during the day?

Most practitioners of the Leangains method find it easier to start the fasting period after dinner, through their sleep and well into the greater part of the next morning.

For example, they eat dinner at 8 in the evening. This also serves for them as a way to socialize with people through having shared dinners.

The fast starts at 9 PM. If they will not sleep immediately, water and other non-caloric beverages are consumed to keep them energized or full.

They wake up at 6 AM and drink coffee or a glass of water. The fasting period is still held. They skip breakfast (probably to do important tasks or go to the gym) and then the next meal would be a heavy brunch at 11AM.

Does this schedule sound familiar?

Most people are already doing this without noticing that they are already following a Leangains fasting-feeding schedule. These people usually include students or office workers who have to hurry early in the morning.

The fasting-feeding schedule of the Leangains method is easy to incorporate into one's lifestyle. Roughly simplified, it means skipping breakfast and taking a good brunch around noon.

However, this schedule should be maintained on a consistent basis in order for it to work on weight loss and muscle building. You should not skip a day on Leangains and have a "cheat day".

This will instantly ruin your progress. You should maintain a 14-hour fast, 6- to 8-hour feeding schedule on a daily basis. If not, then the hormonal response you want to stimulate won't happen.

Fasting period

The body releases hormones that stimulate fat burning during the fasting period. It also decreases insulin levels to allow for maximum energy conversion from the body's fat stores.

However, this does not happen immediately. Sustained practice will trigger these events in the body.

In order for these processes to happen, the body should have a consistent fasting-feeding schedule.

If not, then the hormonal balance and interactions are thrown out of rhythm and maximum fat burning is not achieved.

The success of Leangains also depend on consistency. Once you pick out the hours of your eating and fasting periods, stick to it.

Changing schedules and hours of eating will make adapting to the Leangains program much harder. The body does not know when to start burning fats and when to use energy from food. This confusion will not make hormonal changes consistent. The body works most efficiently if it follows a timetable.

Feeding period

During the feeding period, the kind of food you eat in relation to the workout is very important. Remember that the Leangains method is most recommended for women who already follow a regular exercise schedule.

More carbohydrates should be eaten on exercise days. The calories from these foods would be quickly used during and after your exercise regimen. On your rest days, eat more fats than carbohydrates.

The amount of protein you eat should be high, whether on exercise days or on rest days. Protein consumption depends on how much lean muscles you wish to gain, your gender (men need slightly higher proteins for muscle building than women), age, activity levels and body fat.

This schedule would help you build lean muscles.

Majority of your daily calories should come from whole and unprocessed foods. While counting calories is not an issue with Leangains, you need to get them from healthy and usable sources.

That is, avoid taking empty calories that your body has no use of.

It will just add to your daily calorie count and get converted into fat because the body cannot use it for energy in muscle building or for your daily activities.

Meals are important, but a meal replacement bar or protein shake should do as a meal if you don't have time to prepare and sit down for a regular meal. The point is to get some usable calories during the feeding period.

The Pros of Leangains method

The most attractive feature of this method is the ease of meal preparation.

Most people who try to lose body fat while building lean muscles often have to make careful meal planning and meticulous calorie counting and meal preparation. They also have to time their meals for optimum results.

With the Leangains method, everything is simple and easy. The frequency of taking meals is irrelevant. You don't have to eat 5 to 6 meals a day, every 3 to 4 hours, etc.

In fact, you can eat at any time during the 6- to 8-hour feeding period. You decide when to eat.

Some people find it easier to eat 3 regular meals within this period. Some opt for smaller, more frequent meals. It all depends on you, as long as it is within the time-frame allotted for the feeding period.

The fasting-feeding schedule is done every day. It is easier to incorporate in one's daily schedule, without having to make major changes or adjustments. In fact, you can use Leangains without putting too much thought into it.

The Cons of the Leangains method

The flexibility of the Leangains method is more on "when to eat" and not on "what to eat". There are specific guidelines to follow when choosing the Leangains method.

These food guidelines are uniquely designed for the person's goals, age, body type, exercise regimen and overall activity level.

The nutrition plan is strict in order to achieve optimum muscle gain. This is also a bit difficult for some women to adhere to.

Also, one potential difficulty is the need to cut out at least 1 meal each day. Most people who are used to eating breakfast in the morning, lunch at noon and dinner in the evening may find the 6-or 8-hour feeding period a bit restrictive.

For some, skipping on a meal or two may also make it more difficult to achieve the weekly calorie requirement.

It is also a bit difficult for some to learn to eat bigger meals to get the calorie requirements.

Again, Leangains is most recommended for people who are already dedicated gym rats. The main goal of this IF method is to lose body fat and help build muscles. If these are not your goals, then try the other IF methods and see what suits you.

CHAPTER 4

Alternate-Day IF Method

The alternate-day fasting method is also known as the UpDayDownDay diet or the Alternate-Day diet.

This method is not easier nor more difficult than Leangains. However, this may be preferable or more enjoyable for some dieters.

This IF method was developed by Dr. James Johnson. Like the Leangains, this also has a significant following and a large number of practitioners.

This is most recommended for people who can follow a strict diet and aim for a defined goal weight. If you are into losing weight but not re-composing your figure, then this method will be excellent for you.

How Alternate-Day IF method works?

The goal of this IF method is to promote weight loss and optimum fat burning. This is observed through holding longer fasting periods. If you can fast for longer than 14 or 16 hours, you may try the Alternate-Day If method.

These fasting periods are done on alternating days each week instead of a daily basis. If you intend to have a longer feeding window, you may want to try this method. However, you would also need to be comfortable about longer fasting periods.

For example, you would eat regular meals on a Monday, ending with dinner. You can eat as much as you want according to your appetite.

The fasting period starts after dinner and for the next 24 hours.

That means, no food is consumed from Monday night's dinner until dinnertime on Tuesday. You would only drink non-caloric beverages or relax with your activities, because you have ample time.

On the next morning, Wednesday, regular meals are resumed. You can eat according to the same patterns that you did last Monday. The last meal that you would also have for the day will be your dinner.

The cycle of fasting starts again from Wednesday after dinner until Thursday dinnertime. Breakfast occurs on Friday.

With this schedule, you can still eat at least 1 meal each day while going on longer fasts (24-hour fasting periods). This is great if you would really like experience days as if you were not on a diet.

In a nutshell, this method is simply eating normally for a day, eating very little food the next day and resume normal eating on the third day.

The fasting or low-calorie days does not mean zero food intake at all. This only means limited calorie intake, which should be about 1/5 of the recommended daily consumption.

That is, for a person who is on a 2,000 daily calorie intake, this amount is eaten on normal days.

On alternate fasting days, the intake should only be at 400 calories only. This is equivalent to one simple meal.

During the "Down" days or fasting days, most people find meal replacement and protein shakes very helpful. These are very filling while still remaining within the calorie limitations.

These shakes can be sipped in small amounts all throughout the day to help stave off hunger and any cravings. This is also a convenient way of fasting because true hunger is not felt while taking small sips of the shakes.

Protein shakes can be taken all throughout the diet regimen. However, meal replacements are only recommended during the 1st 2 weeks into the Alternate-Day IF method.

The purpose of incorporating them in the initial periods is simply to help the dieter adjust to the fasting hours.

You will notice that as you on fasts each day or every other day, the next fasting period becomes easier to handle. At this point you may not even to sip shakes all day. A small meal would suffice.

When you incorporate exercise, low calorie days or "down" days are not the best days to schedule your exercise sessions. If you have to train or exercise, opt for lighter sessions. Save the heavier exercise routines on normal eating days.

The Pros of Alternate-Day IF method

One of the main benefits from this IF method is the longer fasting period, compared to that of Leangains.

A longer fasting period is believed to stimulate more fat burning process and faster weight loss. You would also achieve more benefits of the fasted state, as we have mentioned in the beginning.

This method also gives optimum weight loss.

The average weight loss with the Alternate-Day IF method is 2 ½ pounds per week, especially when cutting out 25 to 35% of calorie intake.

On longer fasts, you burn more fat, and you can expect results to become easily visible on a shorter period of time.

Another advantage to the alternate-fasting method is that people can still enjoy their meals because the size and quality remains pretty much the same.

In some days, one can even feast (but not to confuse with binge!). And all these while still losing some weight.

The Cons of Alternate-Day IF method

One of the disadvantages of this IF method is training the body to eat a lot for a day, then go on fast the next day.

This is a radical difference with respect to eating patterns that have been previously followed.

This may be a bit difficult for some, especially those who spent a lifetime of eating average meal portions at regular times each day of the week.

The alternate-day fasting method also requires a bit of careful planning, cooking and consistent eating.

Expect the feeding days to be more hectic than non-feeding days. You should also plan your only meal during the feeding day.

Another potential difficulty is bingeing. Some people tend to overcompensate on the day after the fast.

They binge eat, which counters any calories and fats burned during the fast. When you eat during your feeding days, always eat slowly and listen to your appetite. Learn to identify physical hunger versus emotional hunger.

To solve this problem, track meals ahead of time. That is, you should have a meal plan for the entire week.

This takes a bit of careful planning but will make everything easier and efficient for you.

You should stick to a prepared list of what to eat and what not to eat on normal eating days and fasting periods.

Also, it may help a lot to have meals prepared well in advance to avoid reaching for unhealthy foods once the fast period is over.

Some people find this method working for them. They do not feel too deprived because they get to eat normally and lose weight.

Fasting periods do not mean zero calorie intakes. They still get to eat, only in minimal amounts (400 to 500 calories throughout the fasting days).

Some may find the 24-hour fasting period too limiting. Not to fret, there are still other IF methods you can try.

CHAPTER 5

Warrior Diet

There are other 3 IF methods which include the Warrior diet, the Fat Loss Forever diet and the Eat-Stop-Eat cycle.

They are similar to Leangains and Alternate-Day fasting wherein fasting and feeding periods are designated. Likewise, they have quick weight loss results and lifestyle benefits to the dieter.

All of these methods incorporate fasting periods in varying schedules.

This means that the only difference among them depends on the actual time on the clock in which fasting and feeding windows are followed. The number of hours for feeding and fasting stay the same.

In this chapter, we will focus on the warrior diet, since this is the main method that Fat Loss Forever and Eat-Stop-Eat follow.

WARRIOR DIET

The warrior diet is based on historical fact. The science behind this is more anthropological than medical.

The Warrior diet originated from the belief that warriors in ancient days used to eat similar to the cycle of the intermittent fasting method. In short, they had fasting and feeding periods.

These were not consciously their plans, but rather a consequence of their lifestyle and profession.

If we perform the warrior diet nowadays, it would be easier because our bodies are adaptable or have previously followed this eating cycle.

It should feel more natural to us. We will only be reliving the previous eating patterns of our ancestors.

This IF method was developed by Ori Hofmekler, and is recommended for people who have no trouble following rules and schedules. This is for the "devoted" weight loss dieters.

Take note that fasting for 20 hours each day implies a lot of resisted temptations throughout the day. One should be completely decided that fasting periods are indeed fasting periods.

If weight loss is your number one priority as of the moment, this can be helpful to you. This is also recommendable to people who have very busy schedules and would like to accomplish more through cutting time for food.

How the Warrior diet works

This IF method incorporates a 20-hour fast each day of the week. This is one of the longest fasting periods for a daily regimen.

This is based on the belief that warriors had to be on their feet (either in training, journey or battle) for most of the day.

They only get to sit down for a meal at night, when they set up camp or return to it after training or a battle. And this supposedly happens in a span of four hours.

It is also based on the belief that the body is originally designed for nocturnal eating.

When we eat, a lot of factors affect the appetite and feelings of fullness. One of these is light. Restaurants know this and this accounts for the reason why they prefer to decorate using mellow lights.

Even if we consider the anthropological evidence alone, we will arrive at the same conclusion.

Ancient humans had to hunt for most of the day. Whatever they hunted is served for dinner. You would have to live the lifestyle of our warriors and ancestors, but of course minus the hunting or the training for battles.

Another premise to the warrior diet is that there was so much to do during the day, such as hunting, gathering, travelling or farming, and eating could not have possibly been done in conjunction to these.

Ancient humans had to take advantage of the light of day and the protection it afforded against predators to perform all their tasks.

When the sun goes down, it was no longer safe for them to be up and about. This was the time they could sit down together and enjoy a meal.

For IF followers, the 20-hour fast ends with a large meal at night. The quality and quantity of food is also crucial to achieve the goal weight.

The fasting period means undereating. Of all intermittent fasting methods, this one assures that you cut your caloric intake.

During feeding periods, you can eat a few servings of raw vegetables or fruits and some proteins. You can also have some fresh juice. It should be in small portions, just enough to stimulate and maximize the body's "Fight or Flight" state.

However, you should remember to eat the minimum amount of calories needed in a day and never go below 1500 calories.

A good sign that you have fed well during the feeding period is when you feel energized by what you ate. Therefore, you should focus on the quality of the food that you eat and keep them nutritious. Do not consume junk food and other empty calories.

During the day, the body is mainly run by the sympathetic system, which helps the body to perform its daily tasks.

With the limited calorie intake, the body will search for other energy sources to support the body's energy needs for the day.

Translation: Fat burning. This "Fight or Flight" state also promotes alertness.

Fasting period lasts for 20 hours each day. The remaining 4 hours is reserved for eating. This is often referred to as the "overeating" phase.

This is done at night, when the parasympathetic system starts to kick in and take over the body's activities. Night is intrinsically designed for rest and relaxation, when the body restores its energy and heals itself.

This is also the time when digestion is at its most efficient function. During the day, the body focuses more on using energy for muscle actions like moving around and working.

Only at night does the body get the optimum time to effectively and efficiently digest food.

When eating at night, start the meal with servings of vegetables, followed by proteins and a few servings of fat. Carbohydrates are only eaten when you are still hungry.

This food schedule is necessary in order to properly start the digestive process for optimum food utilization.

This food schedule is pretty much how 3-, 4- or 5-coursemeals are served. An appetizer of vegetable salad starts the meal. A main course of protein, with a few amounts of fat follows. The meal is rounded off with a carbohydrate-based dessert.

The Pros of the Warrior diet

A lot of women find themselves drawn and loving the Warrior diet. The main attraction is that they still get to eat during the fasting periods.

This is also one of the reasons why people choose to follow the standard day-to-day fasting IF method.

The creativity and resourcefulness implied by the importance of a four-hour feeding window also makes people consume more nutritious food and enjoy it on a daily basis.

There are many pre-packed food that is perfect for the warrior diet. These food contains a lot of energy and nutrition for people who are "always on the go".

These small snacks of fruits, proteins and vegetables help to stave off hunger and fight any cravings.

These small snacks also help in keeping the energy and concentration throughout the day. Most followers of the Warrior diet report better concentration, energy levels and productivity, with an increase in fat loss.

The Cons of the Warrior diet

Some people cannot tolerate long fasting periods. Even with the small snacks throughout the day, they still find it difficult to stay on the Warrior diet.

Also, some people may find it much of an effort to follow strict eating guidelines and order of food when eating.

This may also disrupt socialization, especially on dinner parties and events. Having to plan and be conscious of foods to eat may be tricky for some women.

The key to successful weight loss is to find the method that best suits your needs and lifestyle. If one method does not work, try another.

Keep trying until you reach your goal of losing weight and staying healthy.

Bonus Chapter

How to Jumpstart Intermittent Fasting

You have now learned everything that you need to know about intermittent fasting. You may have even chosen the method that best fits your lifestyle.

But how exactly do you incorporate these steps and instructions to your way of living?

This chapter will give you tips on how you can easily adapt to the intermittent fasting method. It will help you adjust and make plans to this new addition to your daily regime.

Tell your family and friends about IF

When going on a weight loss program, tell your friends and family about your choice and how you intend to achieve it.

Most people are worried about telling other people regarding their health and fitness plans. They may be afraid of disappointment or fear that people will keep them constantly under inspection.

They also want to avoid frustration in case they went on a dieting plan but failed to continue it.

If you are doing IF, disregard these unnecessary worries and assert yourself. First of all, you do not have to worry about potential failures; IF is a very efficient weight loss plan.

You would need to tell your friends and family about IF so you can gain support and cooperation from them.

Eating meals and dining is a considerably social activity. If you are going to do IF, you should realize that some of your social activities may be changed because of IF.

Depending on the method that you choose, you may not be able to engage in dining and dinners if they do not fit inside your feeding window.

People will understand these changes in your life when they know that you are committing to IF and weight loss.

Do not come up with promises and excuses. You should be proud of your weight loss plans.

How to say no to food

This invitation may come from yourself or from other people. You can easily explain your IF goals to others, but sometimes your body will not completely listen to you.

Getting used to having several meals a day, you will crave food during the hours when you used to eat.

This is also called emotional hunger. You are not physically hungry or your body has not yet completely burnt energy from your previous meal but you will have a desire to eat.

To deal with this, simply stop thinking about food. If you think about your next meal, you may even feel more emotionally hungry.

Focus yourself on other activities like reading a book or listening activities. Engage in activities that you enjoyed so well, sometimes you bothered skipping a meal just to keep on doing it.

Anticipating the benefits and effects of IF

If you intend to lose a lot of weight, do not hurry the process of your weight loss. There is a safe amount of weight to lose in a week.

If you are not seeing progress fast, you simply have to wait. You do not have to tweak your IF diet or impose grueling rules to your eating.

It normally takes several weeks to see physical changes that are a product of weight loss.

If you started at a lighter weight, the changes even appear slower. Do not obsess on every inch that you should lose or every pound that you should take off. This will only make dieting difficult for you.

What you should do best is to enjoy IF and the benefit that it gives to your life. There are several benefits to the IF other than weight loss, as you have read from the previous chapters.

Take these in mind and let weight loss come naturally, sometimes to your surprise. No morning could be better than when you try to wear an old pair of jeans then suddenly find out that they now fit you.

CONCLUSION

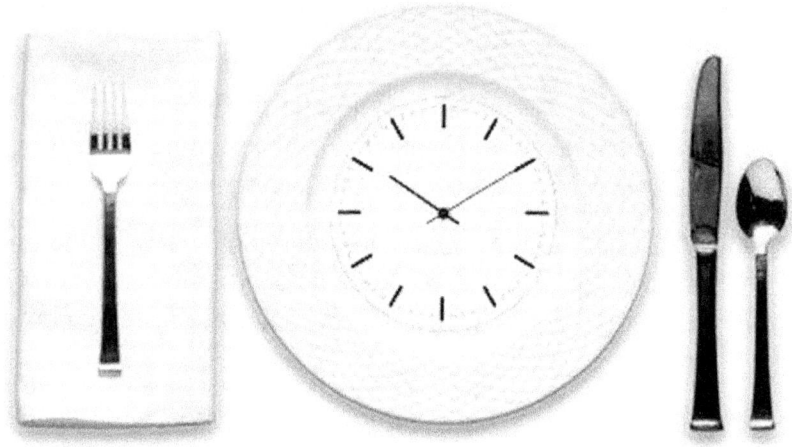

Thank you again for downloading this book!

I hope this book was able to help you to learn all you can about intermittent fasting.

The next step is to start following the steps of the IF method you feel would be best suited for your needs, goals and lifestyle.

Fasting is not necessarily no food intake. You can still eat, but in limited amounts. Keep focused on your goal.

This will help you get past any difficulties you may face. For best results, set your goal before beginning any weight loss regimen and your goal should always include your desire to have a healthier body.

Finally, if you enjoyed this book, then I'd like to ask you for a favor, would you be kind enough to leave a review for this book on Amazon? It'd be greatly appreciated!

Please leave a review for this book on Amazon!

Thank you and good luck!